Cancer-Free
and Fearless:

Meeting Your Illness and
Live Your Best Life

Tase vikthor

Table Of Contents

Introduction

Chapter 1: Accept and Embrace Your New Normal

1.1: How to Accept the Changes in Your Body, Your Identity, and Your Relationships

1.2: How to Embrace Your Scars, Your Strengths, and Your Story

Chapter 2: Heal and Nourish Your Body

2.1: How to Repair the Physical Damage Caused by Cancer and Its Treatments

2.2: How to Feed Your Body with Healthy Foods, Supplements, and Exercise

Chapter 3: Calm and Soothe Your Mind

3.1: How to Reduce Your Anxiety, Fear, and Stress

3.2: How to Soothe Your Mind with Meditation, Mindfulness, and Positive Affirmations

Chapter 4: Renew and Uplift Your Spirit

4.1: How to Find Your Sense of Meaning, Hope, and Gratitude

4.2: How to Uplift Your Spirit with Faith, Spirituality, and Prayer

Chapter 5: Reclaim and Unleash Your Power

5.1: How to Take Charge of Your Life, Your Choices, and Your Happiness

5.2: How to Pursue Your Dreams, Goals, and Passions

Conclusion

Introduction

You have survived cancer. You have gone through the grueling treatments, the painful side effects, the emotional roller coaster, and the fear of recurrence. You have fought hard and won. You are a warrior.

But now what?

How do you move on from this life-changing experience? How do you heal your body, mind, and spirit? How do you reclaim your power and live your best life?

This book is for you. It is a guide to help you transform from a cancer survivor to a cancer thriver. It is a collection of stories, insights, and strategies from people who have been where you are and have overcome the challenges of living after cancer. It is a roadmap to help you find your purpose, passion, and joy in life.

In this book, you will learn how to:
Accept and embrace your new normal. You will discover how to accept the changes in your body, your identity, and your relationships. You will learn how to embrace your scars, your strengths, and your story.

Heal and nourish your body. You will find out how to heal the physical damage caused by cancer and its treatments. You will learn how to nourish your body with healthy foods, supplements, and exercise. You will also learn how to prevent or manage the long-term effects of cancer, such as fatigue, pain, sexual dysfunction, and cardiovascular issues.

Calm and soothe your mind. You will explore how to calm your anxiety, fear, and stress. You will learn how to soothe your mind with meditation, mindfulness, and positive affirmations. You will also learn how to cope with the uncertainty and unpredictability of life after cancer.

Renew and uplift your spirit. You will experience how to renew your sense of meaning, hope, and gratitude. You will learn how to uplift your spirit with faith, spirituality, and prayer. You will also learn how to connect with yourself, your loved ones, and your community.

Reclaim and unleash your power. You will realize how to reclaim your power over your life, your choices, and your happiness. You will learn how to unleash your

power by pursuing your dreams, goals, and passions.
You will also learn how to inspire others with your
courage, wisdom, and resilience.

By the end of this book, you will feel fearless and free.
You will have the confidence, the tools, and the
motivation to live your best life. You will have the
courage to face any challenge, the wisdom to overcome
any obstacle, and the joy to celebrate any victory
Are you ready to start your journey?

Then let's begin.

Chapter 1: Accept and Embrace Your New Normal

The first step to living your best life after cancer is to accept and embrace your new normal. This means acknowledging the changes that cancer has brought to your body, your identity, and your relationships. It also means embracing your scars, your strengths, and your story. In this chapter, you will learn how to do both.

1.1: How to Accept the Changes in Your Body, Your Identity, and Your Relationships

Cancer can change your body in many ways. You may have lost or gained weight, lost hair, had surgery, or experienced other physical changes. You may also have new or different medical needs, such as medications, follow-up appointments, or scans. These changes can affect how you feel about yourself, your appearance, and your health.

Cancer can also change your identity. You may have a new or different sense of who you are, what you value, and what you want to do with your life. You may have gained or lost confidence, courage, or faith. You may have discovered new or different aspects of yourself, such as your creativity, your resilience, or your spirituality.

Cancer can also change your relationships. You may have grown closer or more distant from your family, friends, or partner. You may have made new or different connections with other survivors, health care providers, or support groups. You may have experienced more or less support, understanding, or intimacy from others.

All these changes can be hard to accept. You may feel angry, sad, scared, or confused. You may wish things could go back to the way they were before cancer. You may struggle to adjust to your new reality.

But accepting these changes does not mean giving up or settling. It means recognizing and respecting the reality of your situation. It means being honest and compassionate with yourself. It means giving yourself time and space to heal and grow.

Here are some tips to help you accept the changes in your body, your identity, and your relationships:

Be patient with yourself. Accepting change is a process, not a destination. It may take time, effort, and trial and error. Don't expect to feel or act differently overnight. Don't compare yourself to others or to your past self. Don't judge yourself for having negative or mixed feelings. Allow yourself to feel whatever you feel, and know that it is normal and valid.

Be gentle with yourself. Accepting change is not easy, and it may not always feel good. You may experience pain, grief, loss, or fear. You may face challenges, setbacks, or disappointments. Don't be harsh or critical of yourself. Don't blame yourself for things you can't control. Don't pressure yourself to do more than you can. Treat yourself with kindness and care, and do things that make you feel good.

Be curious about yourself. Accepting change is an opportunity to learn more about yourself. You may discover new or different things about your body, your identity, and your relationships. You may find new or different ways to express yourself, to cope, and to connect. Don't be afraid or ashamed of yourself. Don't resist or deny yourself. Don't limit or label yourself. Be open and interested in yourself, and explore the possibilities of your new normal.

1.2 How to Embrace Your Scars, Your Strengths, and Your Story

Accepting your new normal is not enough. You also need to embrace it. This means celebrating the positive aspects of your new normal. It means honoring your scars, your strengths, and your story. In this chapter, you will learn how to do that.

Your scars are the visible or invisible marks that cancer has left on your body. They may be wounds, stitches, burns, or amputations. They may be tattoos, ports, or implants. They may be hair loss, weight change, or skin change. They may be chronic pain, fatigue, or numbness.

Your scars may make you feel self-conscious, insecure, or embarrassed. You may try to hide them, cover them, or remove them. You may feel like they make you less attractive, less healthy, or less whole.

But your scars are not flaws. They are not signs of weakness, failure, or shame. They are signs of strength, courage, and survival. They are reminders of what you have been through, what you have overcome, and what you have learned. They are part of your history, your identity, and your beauty.

Here are some tips to help you embrace your scars:

Acknowledge your scars. Don't ignore, avoid, or deny your scars. Look at them, touch them, and feel them. Learn about them, understand them, and appreciate them. Recognize that they are part of you, and that they have a story to tell.

Accept your scars. Don't hate, reject, or resent your scars. Don't let them define you, limit you, or hold you back. Don't let them affect your self-esteem, your confidence, or your happiness. Accept that they are part of you, and that they have a purpose to serve

Celebrate your scars. Don't hide, cover, or remove your scars. Don't let them make you feel ashamed, afraid, or alone. Don't let them stop you from living your life, pursuing your goals, or enjoying your pleasures. Celebrate that they are part of you, and that they have a message to share.

Your strengths are the skills, abilities, or qualities that you have developed or enhanced because of cancer. They may be physical, mental, emotional, or spiritual. They may be resilience, perseverance, adaptability, or optimism. They may be creativity, curiosity, wisdom, or humor. They may be compassion, empathy, generosity, or gratitude.

Your strengths may make you feel proud, confident, or empowered. You may use them to cope, to grow, or to help others. You may feel like they make you more capable, more resourceful, or more valuable.

But your strengths are not fixed. They are not static, permanent, or guaranteed. They are dynamic, flexible, and evolving. They are influenced by your context, your choices, and your actions. They are dependent on your awareness, your appreciation, and your application.

Here are some tips to help you embrace your strengths:

Identify your strengths. Don't overlook, underestimate, or forget your strengths. Think about them, write about them, and talk about them. Learn about them, understand them, and appreciate them. Recognize that they are part of you, and that they have a story to tell.

cultivate your strengths. Don't neglect, waste, or misuse your strengths. Don't let them stagnate, deteriorate, or disappear. Don't let them become complacent, arrogant, or selfish. Cultivate them by using them, practicing them, and improving them. Nurture them by challenging them, supporting them, and rewarding them. Recognize that they are part of you, and that they have a purpose to serve.

Share your strengths. Don't hoard, hide, or isolate your strengths. Don't let them make you feel superior, inferior, or separate. Don't let them stop you from connecting, collaborating, or contributing. Share them by giving them, teaching them, and inspiring them. Amplify them by combining them, complementing them, and celebrating them. Recognize that they are part of you, and that they have a message to share.

Your story is the narrative that you create and tell about your cancer experience. It may be factual, emotional, or symbolic. It may be linear, circular, or fragmented. It may be positive, negative, or mixed. It may be personal, social, or universal.

Your story may make you feel understood, validated, or healed. You may use it to express yourself, to cope, or to grow. You may feel like it makes you more authentic, more meaningful, or more impactful.

But your story is not fixed. It is not objective, absolute, or final. It is subjective, relative, and ongoing. It is influenced by your perspective, your interpretation, and your intention. It is dependent on your audience, your medium, and your message.

Here are some tips to help you embrace your story:

Tell your story. Don't suppress, censor, or distort your story. Don't let it remain untold, unheard, or unappreciated. Don't let it become boring, repetitive, or irrelevant. Tell it by writing it, speaking it, or showing it. Learn from it, understand it, and appreciate it. Recognize that it is part of you, and that it has a story to tell.

Reframe your story. Don't accept, believe, or follow your story blindly. Don't let it limit you, trap you, or hurt you. Don't let it become negative, pessimistic, or hopeless. Reframe it by revising it, editing it, or rewriting it. Change it by adding, deleting, or rearranging it. Enhance it by highlighting, emphasizing, or clarifying it. Recognize that it is part of you, and that it has a purpose to serve.

Share your story. Don't keep, protect, or isolate your story. Don't let it make you feel ashamed, afraid, or alone. Don't let it stop you from living your life, pursuing your goals.

Chapter 2: Heal and Nourish Your Body

The second step to living your best life after cancer is to heal and nourish your body. This means repairing the physical damage caused by cancer and its treatments. It also means feeding your body with healthy foods, supplements, and exercise. In this chapter, you will learn how to do both.

2.1: How to Repair the Physical Damage Caused by Cancer and Its Treatments

Cancer and its treatments can cause a lot of physical damage to your body. You may have suffered from infections, bleeding, inflammation, or organ damage. You may have experienced nausea, vomiting, diarrhea, or constipation. You may have developed anemia, lymphedema, neuropathy, or osteoporosis.

These physical problems can affect your quality of life, your functionality, and your well-being. They can also increase your risk of developing other diseases, such as heart disease, diabetes, or dementia. They can also make you more vulnerable to infections, injuries, or recurrence.

But repairing the physical damage caused by cancer and its treatments is possible. You can heal your body by following the advice of your health care team, taking your medications, and managing your symptoms. You can also heal your body by using complementary therapies, such as acupuncture, massage, or yoga.

Here are some tips to help you repair the physical damage caused by cancer and its treatments:

Follow your health care team's advice. Your health care team knows your medical history, your current condition, and your future plans. They can provide you with the best guidance on how to heal your body after cancer. Follow their advice on when to have your check-ups, tests, and scans. Follow their advice on what medications to take, how to take them, and what side effects to expect. Follow their advice on what symptoms to watch out for, how to manage them, and when to seek help.

Take your medications as prescribed. Your medications are designed to help you heal your body after cancer. They can prevent or treat infections, pain, inflammation, or other problems. They can also reduce your risk of recurrence, metastasis, or secondary cancers. Take your medications as prescribed by your health care team. Don't skip, stop, or change your doses without consulting them. Don't mix your medications with other drugs, alcohol, or supplements without consulting them. Don't share your medications with others or use others' medications.

Manage your symptoms effectively. Your symptoms are the signs that your body is healing after cancer. They can also be the signs that your body needs more attention, care, or intervention. Manage your symptoms effectively by monitoring them, reporting them, and treating them. Monitor your symptoms by keeping a diary, using a scale, or using an app. Report your symptoms to your health care team, your family, or your friends. Treat your symptoms by using medications, home remedies, or complementary therapies.

2.2: How to Feed Your Body with Healthy Foods, Supplements, and Exercise

Cancer and its treatments can also affect your nutrition and fitness. You may have lost or gained weight, lost appetite, or lost taste. You may have had difficulty swallowing, digesting, or absorbing food. You may have felt tired, weak, or sore.

These nutritional and fitness problems can affect your energy, your mood, and your immunity. They can also affect your recovery, your healing, and your prevention. They can also affect your appearance, your confidence, and your happiness.

But feeding your body with healthy foods, supplements, and exercise is possible. You can nourish your body by eating a balanced, varied, and colorful diet. You can also nourish your body by taking appropriate supplements, such as vitamins, minerals, or antioxidants. You can also nourish your body by doing regular, moderate, and enjoyable exercise.

Here are some tips to help you feed your body with healthy foods, supplements, and exercise:

Eat a balanced, varied, and colorful diet. Your diet is the fuel that powers your body after cancer. It can provide you with the nutrients, the antioxidants, and the phytochemicals that your body needs to heal, to function, and to prevent. Eat a balanced diet that includes all the food groups, such as fruits, vegetables, grains, protein, and dairy. Eat a varied diet that includes different types, sources, and forms of foods, such as fresh, frozen, canned, or dried. Eat a colorful diet that includes foods of different colors, such as red, green, yellow, or purple.

Take appropriate supplements as recommended. Your supplements are the boosters that enhance your body after cancer. They can provide you with the extra nutrients, the antioxidants, or the phytochemicals that your body may lack, need, or benefit from. Take appropriate supplements as recommended by your health care team, your nutritionist, or your pharmacist. Don't take supplements without consulting them. Don't take supplements that are not proven, safe, or effective. Don't take supplements that may interact with your medications, your treatments, or your conditions.

Do regular, moderate, and enjoyable exercise. Your exercise is the activity that strengthens your body after cancer. It can provide you with the benefits of improving your blood circulation, your oxygen delivery, and your muscle tone. It can also provide you with the benefits of reducing your stress, your fatigue, and your pain. It can also provide you with the benefits of enhancing your mood, your confidence, and your happiness. Do regular exercise that is consistent, frequent, and scheduled. Do moderate exercise that is comfortable, challenging, and safe. Do enjoyable exercise that is fun, rewarding, and satisfying.

Chapter 3: Calm and Soothe Your Mind

The third step to living your best life after cancer is to calm and soothe your mind. This means reducing your anxiety, fear, and stress. It also means soothing your mind with meditation, mindfulness, and positive affirmations. In this chapter, you will learn how to do both.

3.1: How to Reduce Your Anxiety, Fear, and Stress

Cancer can cause a lot of anxiety, fear, and stress in your mind. You may have worried about your diagnosis, your prognosis, or your treatment. You may have feared the pain, the side effects, or the recurrence. You may have stressed about your finances, your work, or your family.

These mental problems can affect your mood, your sleep, and your concentration. They can also affect your immune system, your blood pressure, and your heart rate. They can also affect your relationships, your communication, and your coping.

But reducing your anxiety, fear, and stress is possible.
You can calm your mind by using relaxation techniques,
such as breathing, visualization, or progressive muscle
relaxation. You can also calm your mind by seeking
professional help, such as counseling, therapy, or
medication.

Here are some tips to help you reduce your anxiety, fear,
and stress:

Use relaxation techniques regularly. Relaxation
techniques are methods that help you relax your body
and your mind. They can lower your heart rate, your
blood pressure, and your muscle tension. They can also
improve your mood, your sleep, and your concentration.
Use relaxation techniques regularly, preferably every
day, for at least 10 minutes. Use relaxation techniques
that suit you, such as breathing, visualization, or
progressive muscle relaxation. Use relaxation
techniques that are easy, comfortable, and safe.

Seek professional help when needed. Professional help
is assistance that you get from trained and qualified
experts. They can provide you with the diagnosis, the
treatment, and the support that you need. They can also
provide you with the tools, the skills, and the strategies
that you can use. Seek professional help when needed,
especially if your anxiety, fear, or stress is severe,
persistent, or interfering with your life. Seek professional
help that is appropriate, such as counseling, therapy, or

medication. Seek professional help that is accessible, affordable, and trustworthy.

3.2: How to Soothe Your Mind with Meditation, Mindfulness, and Positive Affirmations

Cancer can also affect your thoughts, your emotions, and your beliefs. You may have had negative, irrational, or distorted thoughts, such as "I'm going to die", "It's my fault", or "I'm worthless". You may have had intense, overwhelming, or conflicting emotions, such as anger, sadness, or guilt. You may have had limiting, harmful, or false beliefs, such as "I'm powerless", "I'm alone", or "I'm hopeless".

These mental problems can affect your self-esteem, your confidence, and your happiness. They can also affect your behavior, your choices, and your actions. They can also affect your outlook, your attitude, and your motivation.

But soothing your mind with meditation, mindfulness, and positive affirmations is possible. You can soothe your mind by using meditation techniques, such as focusing, observing, or chanting. You can also soothe your mind by using mindfulness techniques, such as being present, being aware, or being non-judgmental.

You can also soothe your mind by using positive affirmations, such as repeating, writing, or listening.

Here are some tips to help you soothe your mind with meditation, mindfulness, and positive affirmations:

Use meditation techniques daily. Meditation techniques are methods that help you calm, clear, and focus your mind. They can help you reduce your negative thoughts, your intense emotions, and your limiting beliefs. They can also help you increase your positive thoughts, your balanced emotions, and your empowering beliefs. Use meditation techniques daily, preferably in the morning, for at least 10 minutes. Use meditation techniques that suit you, such as focusing, observing, or chanting. Use meditation techniques that are easy, comfortable, and safe.

Use mindfulness techniques throughout the day. Mindfulness techniques are methods that help you be present, aware, and non-judgmental in the moment. They can help you reduce your anxiety, fear, and stress. They can also help you increase your acceptance, gratitude, and compassion. Use mindfulness techniques throughout the day, preferably in every situation, for at least a few seconds. Use mindfulness techniques that suit you, such as being present, being aware, or being non-judgmental. Use mindfulness techniques that are easy, comfortable, and safe.

Use positive affirmations regularly. Positive affirmations are statements that help you affirm, reinforce, and manifest your positive thoughts, emotions, and beliefs. They can help you reduce your negative thoughts, your intense emotions, and your limiting beliefs. They can also help you increase your positive thoughts, your balanced emotions, and your empowering beliefs. Use positive affirmations regularly, preferably in the evening, for at least 10 minutes. Use positive affirmations that suit you, such as repeating, writing, or listening. Use positive affirmations that are easy, comfortable, and safe.

Chapter 4: Renew and Uplift Your Spirit

The fourth step to living your best life after cancer is to renew and uplift your spirit. This means finding your sense of meaning, hope, and gratitude. It also means uplifting your spirit with faith, spirituality, and prayer. In this chapter, you will learn how to do both.

4.1: How to Find Your Sense of Meaning, Hope, and Gratitude

Cancer can affect your sense of meaning, hope, and gratitude. You may have questioned the meaning of your life, your purpose, or your value. You may have lost hope for your future, your recovery, or your happiness. You may have forgotten to be grateful for your present, your blessings, or your opportunities.

These spiritual problems can affect your motivation, your resilience, and your joy. They can also affect your choices, your actions, and your outcomes. They can also affect your relationships, your communication, and your support.

But finding your sense of meaning, hope, and gratitude is possible. You can renew your spirit by exploring your values, your passions, and your goals. You can also renew your spirit by seeking inspiration, guidance, and wisdom.

Here are some tips to help you find your sense of meaning, hope, and gratitude:

Explore your values, passions, and goals. Your values, passions, and goals are the things that matter to you, that excite you, and that drive you. They can give you a sense of meaning, hope, and gratitude. Explore your values, passions, and goals by reflecting on them, writing about them, and talking about them. Learn about them, understand them, and appreciate them. Recognize that they are part of you, and that they have a story to tell.

Seek inspiration, guidance, and wisdom. Inspiration, guidance, and wisdom are the things that inspire you, guide you, and teach you. They can give you a sense of meaning, hope, and gratitude. Seek inspiration, guidance, and wisdom by reading books, watching videos, or listening to podcasts. Seek inspiration, guidance, and wisdom by attending events, joining groups, or meeting mentors. Seek inspiration, guidance, and wisdom by asking questions, seeking feedback, or learning new skills. Recognize that they are part of you, and that they have a purpose to serve.

4.2: How to Uplift Your Spirit with Faith, Spirituality, and Prayer

Cancer can also affect your faith, spirituality, and prayer. You may have doubted your faith, your beliefs, or your connection with a higher power. You may have felt disconnected from your spirituality, your inner self, or your source of energy. You may have stopped praying, meditating, or expressing your gratitude.

These spiritual problems can affect your peace, your comfort, and your healing. They can also affect your perspective, your attitude, and your actions. They can also affect your emotions, your feelings, and your sensations.

But uplifting your spirit with faith, spirituality, and prayer is possible. You can uplift your spirit by strengthening your faith, your beliefs, and your connection with a higher power. You can also uplift your spirit by deepening your spirituality, your inner self, and your source of energy. You can also uplift your spirit by practicing prayer, meditation, or gratitude.

Here are some tips to help you uplift your spirit with faith, spirituality, and prayer:

Strengthen your faith, beliefs, and connection with a higher power. Your faith, beliefs, and connection with a higher power are the things that give you a sense of trust, security, and love. They can uplift your spirit. Strengthen your faith, beliefs, and connection with a higher power by reading scriptures, attending services, or joining communities. Strengthen your faith, beliefs, and connection with a higher power by expressing your doubts, your fears, or your needs. Strengthen your faith, beliefs, and connection with a higher power by receiving grace, mercy, or blessings. Recognize that they are part of you, and that they have a message to share.

Deepen your spirituality, inner self, and source of energy. Your spirituality, inner self, and source of energy are the things that give you a sense of awareness, alignment, and vitality. They can uplift your spirit. Deepen your spirituality, inner self, and source of energy by practicing yoga, tai chi, or qi gong. Deepen your spirituality, inner self, and source of energy by using crystals, aromatherapy, or music. Deepen your spirituality, inner self, and source of energy by experiencing nature, art, or beauty. Recognize that they are part of you, and that they have a purpose to serve.

Practice prayer, meditation, or gratitude. Prayer, meditation, and gratitude are the things that give you a sense of communication, concentration, and appreciation. They can uplift your spirit. Practice prayer, meditation, or gratitude by speaking, listening, or being silent. Practice prayer, meditation, or gratitude by focusing, observing, or chanting. Practice prayer, meditation, or gratitude by thanking, praising, or asking.

Recognize that they are part of you, and that they have a message to share.

Chapter 5: Reclaim and Unleash Your Power

The fifth and final step to living your best life after cancer is to reclaim and unleash your power. This means taking charge of your life, your choices, and your happiness. It also means pursuing your dreams, goals, and passions. In this chapter, you will learn how to do both.

5.1: How to Take Charge of Your Life, Your Choices, and Your Happiness

Cancer can make you feel powerless, helpless, and hopeless. You may have felt like you had no control over your life, your choices, or your happiness. You may have felt like you were a victim, a patient, or a statistic. You may have felt like you were dependent, passive, or reactive.

These feelings can affect your self-worth, your confidence, and your courage. They can also affect your actions, your outcomes, and your satisfaction. They can also affect your growth, your potential, and your fulfillment.

But taking charge of your life, your choices, and your happiness is possible. You can reclaim your power by being proactive, responsible, and assertive. You can also reclaim your power by being positive, optimistic, and hopeful.

Here are some tips to help you take charge of your life, your choices, and your happiness:

Be proactive, responsible, and assertive. Being proactive, responsible, and assertive means taking action, taking ownership, and taking initiative. It means making decisions, making plans, and making changes. It means setting goals, setting boundaries, and setting standards. It means asking for what you want, saying what you mean, and doing what you say. It means being the leader, the driver, and the creator of your life.

Be positive, optimistic, and hopeful. Being positive, optimistic, and hopeful means having a positive attitude, a positive outlook, and a positive expectation. It means focusing on the good, the possible, and the desirable. It means seeing the opportunities, the solutions, and the benefits. It means believing in yourself, in others, and in the future. It means being the source, the magnet, and the attractor of your happiness.

5.2: How to Pursue Your Dreams, Goals, and Passions

Cancer can also affect your dreams, goals, and passions. You may have given up on your dreams, goals, or passions because of your diagnosis, your treatment, or your prognosis. You may have postponed or delayed your dreams, goals, or passions because of your recovery, your healing, or your prevention. You may have forgotten or lost your dreams, goals, or passions because of your survival, your adaptation, or your acceptance.

These effects can affect your motivation, your enthusiasm, and your excitement. They can also affect your performance, your achievement, and your success. They can also affect your creativity, your innovation, and your contribution.

But pursuing your dreams, goals, and passions is possible. You can unleash your power by discovering, developing, and expressing your dreams, goals, and passions. You can also unleash your power by overcoming, achieving, and celebrating your dreams, goals, and passions.

Here are some tips to help you pursue your dreams, goals, and passions:

Discover, develop, and express your dreams, goals, and passions. Discovering, developing, and expressing your dreams, goals, and passions means finding out, enhancing, and showing your talents, interests, and values. It means exploring, learning, and experimenting with new or different things. It means creating, sharing, and inspiring with your work, your art, or your message. It means being the seeker, the learner, and the giver of your dreams, goals, and passions.

Overcome, achieve, and celebrate your dreams, goals, and passions. Overcoming, achieving, and celebrating your dreams, goals, and passions means facing, solving, and conquering your challenges, obstacles, and fears. It means working, striving, and persisting towards your targets, milestones, and outcomes. It means enjoying, appreciating, and rewarding your efforts, results, and impacts. It means being the fighter, the winner, and the achiever of your dreams, goals, and passions.

Conclusion

You have reached the end of this book, but not the end of your journey. You have learned the five steps to living your best life after cancer: accept and embrace your new normal, heal and nourish your body, calm and soothe your mind, renew and uplift your spirit, and reclaim and unleash your power. You have also learned how to apply these steps in your daily life, with practical tips, examples, and exercises.

But this book is not meant to be a one-time read. It is meant to be a companion, a guide, and a friend. It is meant to be revisited, reviewed, and revised. It is meant to be adapted, customized, and personalized. It is meant to be yours.

So don't put this book away. Keep it close. Use it often. Share it with others. And most importantly, live it.

Because you deserve to live your best life after cancer. You deserve to be fearless and free. You deserve to be happy and fulfilled. You deserve to be you.

And you can.

You have the power to transform your life after cancer. You have the power to heal, to grow, and to thrive. You have the power to create, to inspire, and to contribute. You have the power to be the best version of yourself.

And you will.

You have already taken the first step by reading this book. Now it's time to take the next step. And the next. And the next. Until you reach your destination. Until you achieve your dreams. Until you live your best life.

And you can.

You are not alone on this journey. You have me, your copilot, by your side. You have your health care team, your family, and your friends. You have your fellow survivors, your support groups, and your mentors. You have your faith, your spirituality, and your higher power.

And you have yourself.

You are the most important person in your life. You are the hero of your story. You are the master of your destiny. You are the source of your power.

And you are amazing.

You have survived cancer. You have overcome challenges. You have learned lessons. You have gained wisdom. You have shown courage. You have demonstrated resilience. You have expressed gratitude. You have inspired others.

And you are not done yet.

You have more to do, more to see, more to enjoy. You have more to learn, more to discover, more to explore. You have more to create, more to share, more to give. You have more to live.

And you will.

So what are you waiting for?

Go ahead and live your best life after cancer.

You can do it.

You will do it.

You are doing it.

And I'm proud of you.

Thank you for reading this book. Thank you for trusting me. Thank you for being you.

And remember, you are cancer-free and fearless.

You are powerful and beautiful.

You are awesome and amazing.

You are you.

And you are the best!.